HEMSROCK J

Conquer: The Five Pillars to Optimal Health

Discover how to achieve optimal health by making changes to five key areas in your life without spending a dime on expensive supplements.

Contents

1

Introduction

When I navigate through the endless stream of information on the internet, from blogs and YouTube to podcasts, I'm often surprised by the sheer volume of 'special hacks' promising to elevate our health to the next level. Whether it's the latest supplement guaranteeing laser focus, boundless energy for daily tasks, or the promise of the best sleep you've ever had. Social media bombards us with a myriad of choices, leading to an overload that often breeds anxiety rather than solutions. While there's some truth in these claims, the reality is that they often fall short for many people. I call these quick-fix supplements to putting a band-aid on a wound: they might provide temporary relief, but they don't address the root of the issue.

So, why did I decide to write this book? My inspiration came from an unlikely source — not a new supplement or a groundbreaking hack, but a tweet by Dr. Andrew Huberman, whose words resonated deeply with me. He spoke about the transformative power of behavioral changes every day can help us achieve robust levels of physical and mental fitness.

In this book, I'll guide you through five key areas which significantly enhance your health. These areas are:

- Sleep
- Exercise
- Nutrition
- Sunlight
- Social Connection

At the end of each chapter, I've included actionable items for you to implement. This is important because, without action, reading this book won't change anything. You might as well continue doing what you've been doing. But if you do take these steps, I assure you, you'll feel a noticeable improvement. For some, the results might be quick; for others, it might take time, but they will come. It took me about five months to consistently adhere to my sleep schedule. I was all over the place with everything and not prioritizing things as they came by.

One mindset hack that has helped me in building consistency to follow through is remembering the one percent rule. I first encountered this rule in the book "Atomic Habits" by James Clear. He reminds us to think about making one percent improvement every day. Over a period, your efforts are going to compound, and you will get the results. One of the reasons people fail to get results is because they do not take action consistently. They expect immediate results and when they don't get it, they give up.

Think of these five areas as foundations for healthier living. If you improve even one, you will see the benefits. If you decide to work on all these slowly with time, you will be way ahead in your health and fitness. Some of you might even feel much better than when they were young.

Embrace this journey with an open mind and a commitment to action.

The path to a healthier, more fulfilling life is right in front of us — and it doesn't require expensive supplements or unconventional hacks. Let's begin this transformative journey together.

2

Sleep

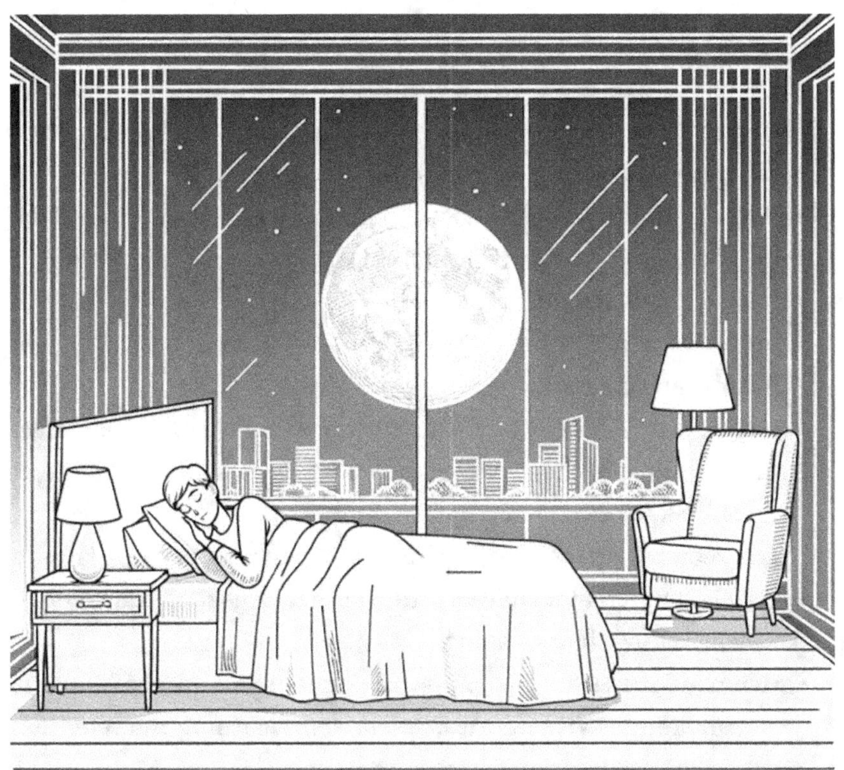

Sleep is a vital process that allows your mind and body to recover. In our fast-paced world, sleep often takes a backseat in our list of priorities. However, understanding the science behind sleep and its profound impact on our well-being can change the way we view those precious hours of rest. This chapter isn't about complex neurological studies; it's about breaking down the essence of sleep in a way that's easy to grasp and apply in our daily lives.

What Happens in Your Body When You Sleep

- **Muscle recovery:** Sleep supports critical bodily functions, such as muscle growth, tissue repair, protein synthesis, etc.
- **Better immunity:** Sleep boosts the immune system and helps the body fight illness. People who don't get enough sleep are at a higher risk of colds and other infections.
- **Cognitive functioning:** Good sleep enhances focus, decision-making, and creativity.
- **Weight loss:** The body regulates hormones during sleep that affect hunger and appetite. People who do not get enough sleep are at higher risk for weight gain.
- **Skin repair:** Sleep affects the skin's ability to recover from damage. A study found that people who regularly fall short of sleep tend to have increased signs of aging.
- **Memory formation:** Sleep plays a pivotal role in processing and consolidating new memories, essential for learning and retention averting the risk of memory loss and dementia.
- **Optimal learning:** The brain forms new pathways during sleep that help with learning and retaining new information. Sleep also improves problem-solving skills, attention, and creativity.
- **Emotional regulation:** Adequate sleep is crucial for maintaining emotional stability and mental health. A lack of sleep makes it harder to enjoy positive experiences and we are relatively more impulsive to deal with situations.
- **Reduces chronic health conditions:** Getting good quality sleep can reduce the risk of chronic diseases cardiovascular diseases, diabetes, obesity, etc.

How Much Sleep Do You Need

The amount of sleep you need varies depending on several factors, including age, health, and lifestyle. Below are the general guidelines as mentioned on the CDC's website:

Age Group	Recommended Hours of Sleep per Day
Newborn 0-3 months	14–17 hours (National Sleep Foundation)[1] No recommendation (American Academy of Sleep Medicine)[2]
Infants 4-12 months	12–16 hours per 24 hours (including naps)[2]
Toddler 1-2 years	11–14 hours per 24 hours (including naps)[2]
Preschool 3-5 years	10–13 hours per 24 hours (including naps)
School Age 6-12 years	9–12 hours per 24 hours
Teens 13-18 years	8–10 hours per 24 hours
Adults 18-60 years 61-64 years 65 years and older	7 or more hours per night 7-9 hours 7-8 hours

Remember, quality of sleep is just as important as quantity. If you have poor sleep quality, then even after sleeping for enough hours, you won't feel well-rested. In the next section, I'm going to share some practical steps which will aid in improving your sleep quality.

How to Get Quality Sleep

Imagine your body as a vehicle: without timely oil changes, the air in the tires, or engine tune-ups, it starts to fail and wear down. Like that, our bodies need more than just sleep - quality sleep. Excellent sleep habits are the key to unlocking this rejuvenating rest. Here are some actionable items to enhance your sleep:

- **Follow a consistent sleep schedule:** Practice going to bed and waking up at the same time every day, even on weekends. This helps regulate your body's clock. After a while, getting up at the same time will become effortless.

- **Control worries before bedtime**: Sleeping without worries enables your mind and body to essentially go through all stages of sleep effectively which contributes to positive sleep quality.

- **Create a restful environment:** Transform your bedroom into a haven for sleep. Make it clean and clutter-free. Keep a cool, dark, and tranquil atmosphere. Consider using earplugs, eye shades, or white noise machines if needed.

- **Limit exposure to electronic devices before bedtime:** Screens emit blue light which interferes with our ability to get proper sleep. Plan to turn off your phone about two hours before you go to bed.

- **Have a bedtime routine:** Develop a bedtime ritual to signal your body it's time to wind down. This could include reading, journaling, meditation, or deep breathing exercises.

- **Stay physically active:** Regular physical activity can promote better sleep. Even just going for a walk helps. Although, try to avoid vigorous workouts close to bedtime.

- **Avoid having food or alcohol too close to bedtime:** Avoid heavy meals, caffeine, and alcohol close to bedtime, as they can disrupt sleep.

While this is not an exhaustive list, there are more than enough to help someone achieve quality sleep. Observe how your body feels as you make changes to your sleep routine. Even after acting on the above items, if you still find that you are not getting quality sleep, consult a sleep doctor. They possess a variety of techniques to identify any sleep disorders if you have one, ultimately aiding you in achieving restful sleep.

3

Exercise

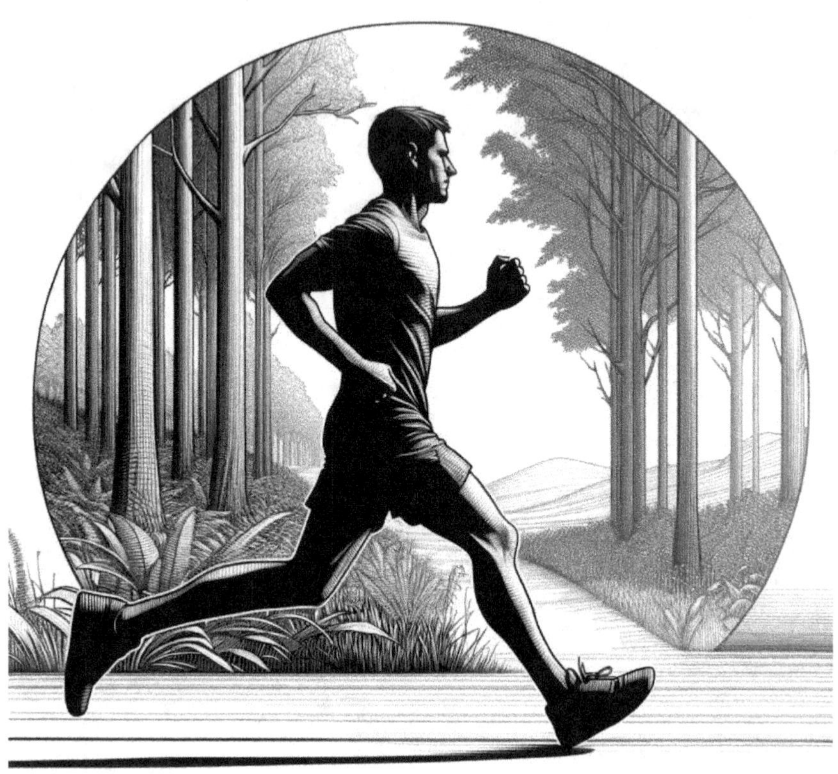

The history of human lifestyle has seen a dramatic transformation, especially in the context of physical activity and fitness. Our early ancestors led an inherently active life. Their survival involved constant physical engagement: hunting, gathering, running from predators, and moving from one place to another. This lifestyle ensured that their bodies were regularly exercised, contributing to robust physical health and fitness. Daily life was their natural gym.

Fast forward to the post-industrialization era and into the digital age, and the contrast couldn't be more evident. The advent of desk jobs and technological advancements has led to a sedentary lifestyle and a significant decrease in physical activity. Most modern-day tasks are accomplished with minimal physical exertion, often just a few clicks or taps away. This shift has profound implications for our physical and mental health. This lack of physical activity is leading to a weakening of bones, decreasing muscle strength and bone density. It's also a major contributor to the rise in chronic diseases like obesity, heart disease, diabetes, etc. There's been a significant uptick in mental health issues like stress, anxiety, and depression as well.

It's a wake-up call to recognize the importance of integrating physical activity back into our daily lives, emulating in some ways the active lifestyle of our ancestors for better health and well-being.

Physical Benefits of Exercising

Exercise triggers a multitude of beneficial processes in our body, contributing significantly to our overall health and fitness. Here's a detailed look at what happens physically when we engage in regular exercise:

- **Muscle building and toning:** Exercise, especially strength training, leads to muscle hypertrophy, where muscle fibers grow and strengthen. Not only do you look good, but also enhances metabolic rate and overall strength.
- **Fat loss:** Physical activity increases the body's energy expenditure, helping to burn stored fat.
- **Joint health improvement:** Regular movement helps maintain joint flexibility and can reduce pain and stiffness, which is particularly beneficial for conditions like arthritis.
- **Enhanced heart health:** Exercise reduces the risk of heart disease by

strengthening the heart muscles, and improving its ability to pump blood efficiently.

- **Improved respiratory efficiency:** Regular exercise enhances lung capacity and efficiency, enabling better oxygen intake and utilization.
- **Bone density increase:** Exercise which involves lifting heavy weights stimulates bone formation and slows down bone density loss, which is crucial for preventing osteoporosis.
- **Promotes better sleep:** Regular physical activity improves the quality of your sleep and also helps falling asleep faster.
- **Stabilizing blood sugar levels:** Regular exercise helps regulate blood sugar concentration, reducing the risk of type 2 diabetes.
- **Healthy digestive system:** Exercise improves gastrointestinal function, reducing the risk of constipation and other digestive disorders.
- **Enhanced immune function:** Regular exercise boosts the immune system, making the body more effective at fighting off infections.
- **Hormonal balance:** Exercise influences the release of various hormones, including endorphins (which improve mood) and hormones that regulate appetite.

Mental Health Benefits of Exercising

Exercise not only transforms our physical health but also has profound effects on our mental well-being. Here are some of the key mental health benefits:

- **Mood enhancement:** Exercise stimulates the release of endorphins, often referred to as 'feel-good' hormones, which naturally boost mood and create a sense of happiness and euphoria.

- **Stress reduction:** Physical activity helps in lowering the body's stress hormones, such as cortisol and adrenaline, leading to a feeling of relaxation and reduced anxiety.
- **Improved cognitive function:** Regular exercise enhances brain functions like memory, attention, and processing speed, primarily due to increased blood flow and oxygen to the brain.
- **Increased self-esteem and confidence:** Achieving exercise goals or improvements in physical appearance can significantly boost self-esteem and overall confidence.
- **Better sleep quality:** Regular physical activity promotes more restful and deeper sleep, which is crucial for mental health, cognitive function, and overall mood.
- **Depression alleviation:** Exercise is a powerful antidote for combating depression, offering natural and effective relief for these common mental health issues.
- **Enhanced brain resilience:** Regular exercise contributes to neuroplasticity, which enhances the brain's ability to adapt and recover from stress and trauma.
- **Social interaction and connectivity:** Group exercises or sports can provide social benefits, reducing feelings of loneliness and isolation and fostering a sense of community.
- **Increased creativity:** Physical activity, especially in a natural setting, can stimulate creativity, providing a mental break and allowing for the incubation of new ideas.

The list goes on and on, but you get the idea. Understanding these physical and mental benefits can be a powerful motivator to incorporate regular exercise into our daily routines, ultimately leading to a healthier, happier, and more balanced life.

What Kind of Exercises You Can Do

If you already incorporated exercise into your daily life, congratulations you are already on the journey to better living. For those of you who don't have any exercise routine, or don't have any idea where to start, here are some of the things you can do:

- Cycling
- Brisk walking
- Swimming
- Running
- Lifting weights
- Stretching
- Dance classes
- Pilates
- Yoga
- Meditation
- Hiking
- Playing sports like Tennis, Pickleball, Basketball, Soccer
- Yard work (mowing, raking)

For some of you, it may seem too much commitment to integrate these changes. I understand and we all have different situations in our lives. If this feels too much, start with walking. Even a fifteen-minute walk every day is great. Remember the mindset I shared with you at the beginning of the book. Focus on one percent improvement every day. Take small steps. Over a period, it will become easier to follow through and make it a habit. Remember, any movement is better than none — the important thing is to get started and keep going

4

Nutrition

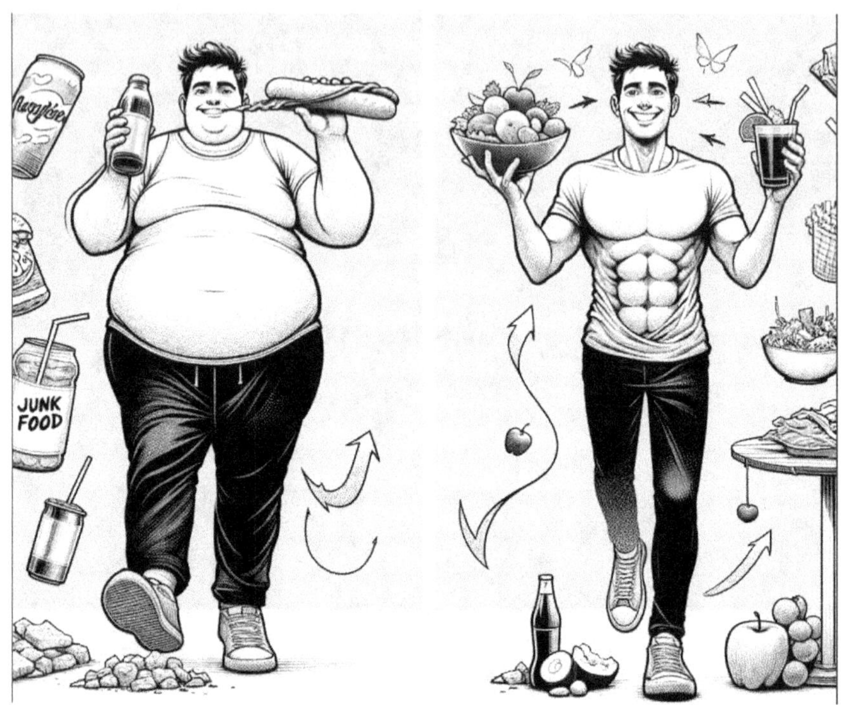

Nutrition plays a vital role in how different body systems and complex processes operate. Food, at its core, is our primary source of energy. This energy is vital for everything from cellular processes to the maintenance of our entire bodily system.

Good nutrition is like providing high-quality fuel for a machine. It ensures that our body functions optimally. This means a robust immune system capable of warding off viruses and diseases, and a well-functioning brain, crucial for everything from daily tasks to complex problem-solving. Conversely, poor nutrition can lead to a gradual yet significant breakdown of bodily functions. The consequences are manifold: increased fatigue due to inefficient energy production, a compromised immune system more susceptible to infections, and an acceleration of the aging process. Additionally, poor nutrition can lead to hormonal imbalances, affecting everything from mood to metabolism.

Thus, the food we consume doesn't just satisfy hunger — it fundamentally influences how we function, feel, and even think. As we delve deeper into this chapter, we'll explore how healthy nutrition is responsible for running different processes in our body. After that, we will talk about eating tips for healthy living.

The Power of Nutrition in Our Biological Processes

Let's investigate how the food we eat has an impact on different processes in our body:

- **Energy production:** The human body uses molecules held in the fats, proteins, and carbohydrates we eat or drink as sources of energy to make ATP (adenosine triphosphate), the energy currency of the cell.
- **Growth and repair:** Proteins from food are essential for the growth and repair of body tissues, including muscles, skin, and organs. After injury or exercise, protein aids in repairing muscle fibers and other tissues.
- **Immune function:** Various nutrients, such as vitamins A, C, and E, and minerals like zinc and selenium, support the immune system. Vitamin C enhances the production of white blood cells, which helps in fighting infections and diseases.
- **Brain function**: Foods rich in omega-3 fatty acids, antioxidants, and vitamins support brain health and cognitive functions. Omega-3s, found in fish, are crucial for brain development and function and may help in managing mood disorders.
- **Hormonal balance:** Fats are responsible for producing & regulating

hormones. Cholesterol is vital for hormone production (including testosterone and estrogen), vitamin D, and bile in the liver (used for food digestion).

- **Digestive health:** Fiber in food helps in maintaining gut health and regular bowel movements. Soluble fiber, found in oats and apples, aids in digestion and can prevent constipation.
- **Bone health:** Calcium and vitamin D from food are crucial for bone strength and density. Dairy products are a primary source of calcium, which is essential for bone health, particularly in children and the elderly.
- **Heart health:** Healthy fats, such as monounsaturated and polyunsaturated fats, support heart health by managing cholesterol levels. Olive oil and nuts contain healthy fats that can help lower the risk of heart disease.
- **Metabolism**: Vitamin B plays a key role in cellular health, growth of red blood cells, brain function, digestion, energy levels, etc. Milk, cheese, eggs, nuts, beans, tuna, whole grains, and cereals are good sources of Vitamin B.
- **Fluid and electrolyte balance:** Electrolytes in food, such as sodium, potassium, and magnesium, help regulate fluid balance and nerve function. Bananas, beans, lentils, etc. are high in potassium, which helps maintain electrolyte balance and prevent muscle cramps.

Set Yourself for Success With Healthy Eating

Adopting healthy eating habits is a crucial step towards achieving your health goals. It's not just about choosing the right foods but also about developing a sustainable approach to nutrition. Here are some habits, tracking methods, and actionable steps you can take to ensure success in your healthy eating journey:

- **Create SMART goals:** Define clear, attainable goals related to your nutrition. Whether it's eating more vegetables, cutting down on sugar, or cooking at home more often, specific goals can guide your food choices.

- **Plan your meals:** Meal planning is a powerful tool. It helps you control what you eat, reduces the likelihood of impulsive unhealthy choices, and can be a time and money saver. Plan your meals weekly and include a variety of nutrient-rich foods.

- **Keep a food diary:** Track what you eat using a food diary or a mobile app. This will help you become more aware of your eating habits and identify areas where you can make healthier choices. There are many free apps that you can download on your phone giving you features for tracking your food intake, and goal setting.

- **Understand portion sizes:** Educate yourself about portion sizes to avoid overeating. Measuring cups, jars, spoons, etc. are very helpful in tracking food quantity.

- **Cook more at home:** Cooking at home gives you control over ingredients and cooking methods, making it easier to eat healthily. Experiment with recipes and cooking techniques to make nutritious meals that you enjoy.

- **Mindful eating:** Practice mindful eating by paying attention to the food you eat, savoring each bite, and listening to your body's hunger and fullness signals. Avoid using TV and phone while having food. This can prevent overeating and enhance your relationship with food.

- **Limit processed foods:** Gradually reduce your intake of processed and high-sugar foods and replace them with whole, unprocessed foods whenever possible.

- **Stay hydrated:** Drink plenty of water throughout the day to stay hydrated and support overall health.

- **Shop wisely:** Make a grocery list before shopping and stick to it. This helps in resisting the temptation to buy unhealthy foods.

- **Seek accountability:** Share your goals with friends or family members who can offer support. Consider joining a group or community focused on healthy eating for motivation and accountability.
- **Be flexible and forgive yourself:** It's okay to have indulgences occasionally. A healthy eating plan is about balance, not perfection.
- **Celebrate your successes:** Recognize and celebrate your achievements, no matter how small. This will help keep you motivated and committed to your healthy eating goals.

By understanding how nutrition affects every aspect of our physical and mental health, and by following these practical tips, you can create a positive, sustainable relationship with food that supports your overall health and well-being.

5

Sunlight

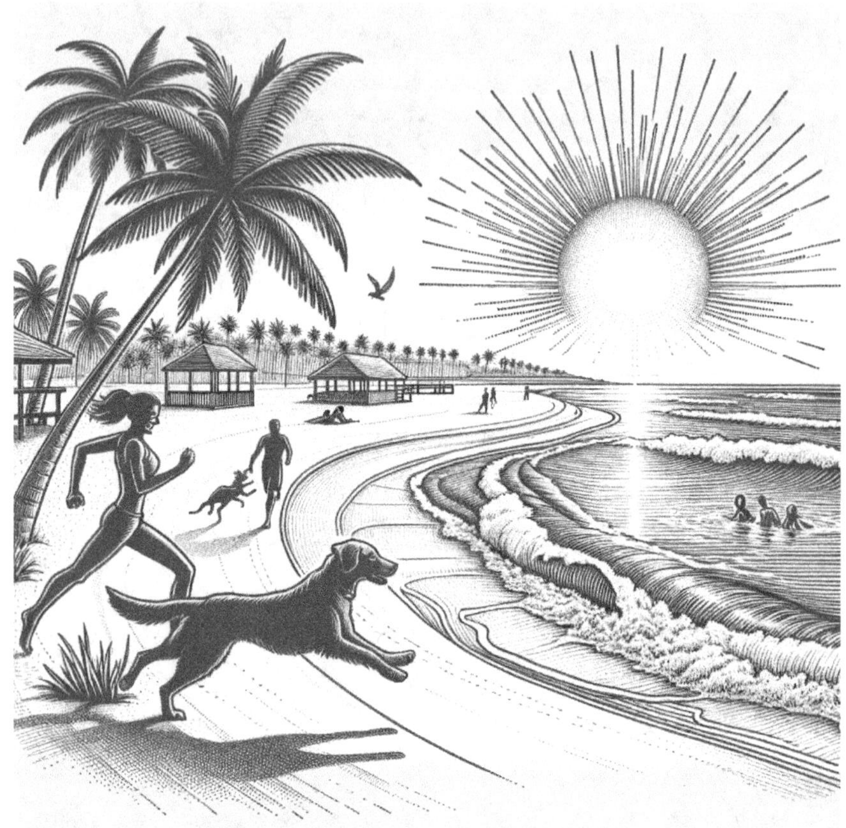

Sunlight is the source and energy for life on this planet. We constantly hear about how too much sun rays can be harmful to the skin. Too much ultraviolet radiation from sun exposure can lead to detrimental effects such as skin damage and even cancer. However, it still stands that humans need a certain degree of it to maintain good health.

In this digital age, a lot of humans spend time working from their desks. And then, they go home only to sit in front of the TV watching their next favorite show. For entertainment, kids prefer to play games on their phones or gaming consoles. Everything is now available in the comfort of our home so the need to go out has diminished causing a lack of exposure to sunlight. Lack of sunlight causes insufficient levels of Vitamin D, mental health disorders, weakened bones, irregular sleep patterns, compromised immune system, etc.

Therefore, it has become increasingly important to incorporate some outdoor time into our daily routines. This may involve setting up fixed time spent doing outdoor activities like playing sports, running, walking hiking, etc. to maintain overall well-being.

I have personally experienced the great benefits of getting sunlight first thing in the morning and it's now part of my morning ritual. As someone who has gone through mood fluctuations throughout my life, this has been a huge blessing to my mental health. I'm honestly addicted to this feeling. I leave my house within thirty minutes of getting up and spend some time running and walking. It supercharges my brain with positivity and puts me in a state to get things accomplished for the day.

The Healing Rays: Sunlight's Role in Physical and Mental Wellness

There are several health benefits associated with getting adequate sunlight:

- **Vitamin D production**: Exposure to sunlight leads to the production of Vitamin D, which is responsible for hormone regulation, healthy bones, a strong immune system, etc.
- **Emotional well-being:** Getting good amounts of sunlight increases levels of serotonin in the brain which is responsible for inducing feelings of happiness, healing wounds, and lowering the risk of

depression and anxiety.

- **Sleep regulation:** Sunlight helps in regulating circadian rhythms which is responsible for deeper and more restful sleep. It also helps in producing melatonin which is a chemical responsible for putting the body into slumber.
- **Weight management:** Getting early exposure to the sun in the morning is believed to help in weight loss. When you have sufficient levels of nutrients, sleep well, and are overall happy, your weight loss efforts are more successful.
- **Stronger bones:** Sun exposure helps the body generate Vitamin D, which in turn builds stronger bones. Vitamin D deficiency causes rickets in children. In adults, it can cause Osteoporosis.
- **Eye health:** A healthy amount of exposure to sunlight is reported to make it less likely to have problems seeing things at a distance. However, it's crucial to avoid too much sun and never look directly at it to prevent eye damage.
- **Lower Blood Pressure:** When sunlight hits the skin, the body releases nitric oxide in the blood which is responsible for lower blood pressure, which reduces the risk of cardiac diseases and stroke thereby improving heart health.

How Much Sunlight You Should Get

The short answer to this is that it's different for everyone. It depends on your skin tone, age, health history, diet, and where you live. In general, anything about 10 and 30 minutes is about right to get the most out of it without causing any health problems. Those with darker skin may require a bit more time in the sun to ensure they are getting enough Vitamin D. You can stay out longer and get the same effect if you use sunscreen. Consult your doctor about what's right for you.

Things You Can Do to Get More Sunlight

- Set a schedule time for going out on walks if you are working in the office or at home. Even going out after lunch for fifteen minutes is great. It also allows you to reset your brain and get back to work more focused.
- If you're an early bird, make it a point to spend at least fifteen minutes in the morning sun. Going up for an early morning workout or run is the best if it fits your schedule.
- Take part in sports which allow you to be outside in nature.
- Cut down exposure to phones and TV during the latter half of the day and instead spend time outside.
- If you have to commute to someplace nearby, switch to walking or biking.
- Plan social activities or pick up hobbies.

We must avoid the risk of overexposure by using sunscreen, shades, etc. so that we can reap the physical and psychological benefits of sunlight.

6

Social Connections

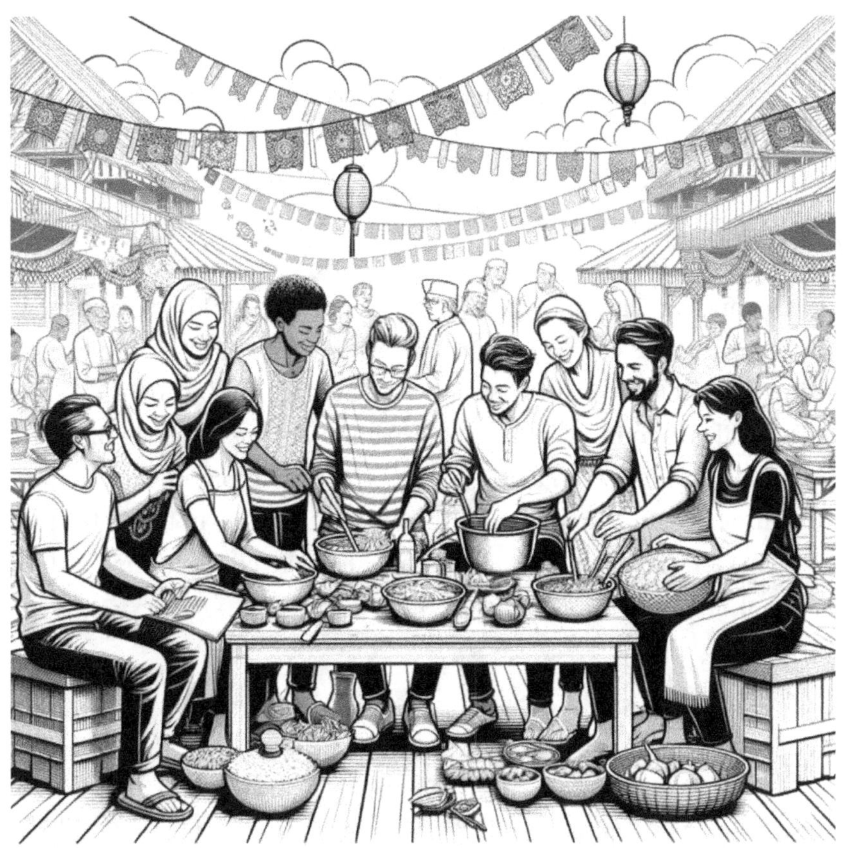

Human beings are hard-wired to be social creatures. Social connections are important for our survival, and we can trace it back to the time when we traveled, and hunted in groups. The chances of surviving for someone who separated from the tribe were quite slim.

While we no longer need to hunt and constantly look for any dangers for our survival in the modern world, having a healthy social connection plays a huge role in our psychological well-being. This applies more to us living in a post-pandemic world. When Covid-19 began, it disrupted life in unforeseen ways which caused people to struggle with isolation, anxiety, and depression. Strict lockdowns were enforced around the world restricting our movement. Not only did it sever our connection with people, but it did so with nature as well which provides us with immense physical and psychological benefits.

Social connections are crucial for our identity, and skill development for prospering in a complex environment. A sense of social connection is increasingly important in today's isolated world. Our relationships with family, friends, coworkers, and community members significantly influence our health and well-being. From the moment we are born till our death; our reliance on others is vital. This is not only true for humans; animals and birds also establish social connections for their survival as well as their young ones.

We Are Hard-Wired to Connect

Matthew D. Lieberman, a professor of psychology at the UCLA College of Letters and Science and a professor of psychiatry and biobehavioral science at UCLA's Semel Institute for Neuroscience and Human Behavior says " Being socially connected is our brain's lifelong passion. It's been baked into our operating system for tens of millions of years."

According to his book "Social: Why Our Brains Are Wired to Connect" when we are not doing anything, our brain tends to think about social connections and our relationships with other people. Our brain has what it's called a 'default network', which is predisposed to social cognition. We are equipped with tools to understand social affairs, minds, and thoughts of other people.

Infants embody this deep need to stay connected from the moment they are born. Among mammals, human babies require prolonged parental care for survival, relying heavily on their mothers. This dependency is highlighted when an infant feel threatened by their mother's absence, as their cries instinctively prompt a maternal response to fulfill their needs. This intricate relationship is a key element in human evolution. This evolution ensures that parental behaviors, such as responding to an infant's cries, are not only necessary for the child's survival but also inherently rewarding for the caregiver, reinforcing the deep-rooted nature of these social bonds.

You need social connections and relationships to survive and thrive. The human brain is built to crave social, and emotional bonds and connection; it feels pain and pleasure based on what is going on socially in your life. Social connections are just as fundamental as sleep, and having food and we tend to suffer if this need is not met. We experience 'social pain'. Neuroimaging research has demonstrated that experiences of social exclusion predominantly activate the dorsal anterior cingulate cortex (dACC) and anterior insula (AI) — regions known to have a role in the distressing experience of physical pain.

How Being Social Impacts Our Physical and Mental Health

- **Improved mental health:** Having strong social connections reduces the risk of depression, anxiety, and overall feelings of loneliness.
- **Building deep relationships:** Oxytocin aka "love hormone" plays a significant role in social bonding and connection. It's released during positive social interactions like hugging, having sex with your partner, etc. thereby promoting feelings of trust, empathy, and connectedness.

- **Increased happiness:** Social People tend to be more confident and exhibit high self – esteem which contributes to their overall happiness.
- **Keeps memory sharp:** Engaging in social interactions tends to lower the risks of dementia as we age.
- **Better health and fitness:** Participating in social gatherings, group activities or community work boosts your physical fitness too. They help reduce the risk of obesity, inflammation, and high blood pressure. Regularly engaging yourself with quality social time tends to build better habits, including watching less TV and other screen time.
- **Enhanced immune system:** Having regular social interactions boosts your immune system, helping the body to fight illness effectively.
- **Low risk of suicide:** Being social helps people to seek the support of friends and family to help them move through challenging situations making them less prone to suicidal tendencies.
- **Improved sleep quality:** Being lonely has been proven to disrupt the quality of sleep, making you feel more fatigued to perform your work and daily routines.

How Can You Be More Social

- **Join a group class:** Various types of group classes can allow you to connect with people having similar interests like dancing, cooking, yoga, meditation, etc.
- **Work at a public place:** Remote work has opened doors to work from anywhere in the world. While it brought a great number of benefits, it has its disadvantages as well. Working from home can make you

feel isolated. Working from a coffee shop, or a library allows you to be surrounded by people.

- **Socialize at work:** Take time to talk to colleagues in the office. Not only do you get to know them better, but it can also open the door for any career opportunities.
- **Host event:** Host an event once a month where you invite your friends or family together just to have a good time.
- **Travel:** If you are not a shy person, traveling allows you to meet people from different parts of the world exposing you to new cultures which helps with confidence, openness, communication skills, building new friendships, etc. thereby contributing to your personal growth.
- **Take part in sports:** Playing sports is an amazing way to connect with people.
- **Volunteer:** Offer your time to charitable or community organizations.
- **Call at least one person a day:** Call someone you haven't talked to in a while. Or call a friend you are close with. Simply talking to someone for five minutes can boost your mood.

If you find yourself feeling disconnected, lonely, and hooked to TV or social media, use that opportunity to remind yourself to stay connected with your friends and families. The psychological benefits of being social are immense and its need cannot be more emphasized in today's world.

7

Conclusion

I hope by reading this book, it inspires you to take action to become healthier and get more out of your life. By embracing these new habits, our bodies can reap these amazing benefits to both physical and mental health. Regardless of your age, with consistent action, patience, and tracking your progress, you will see remarkable improvements in your health. I'll leave you with this Arabian Proverb to ponder –

"He who has health has hope; and he who has hope, has everything."

If you found the material inside this book helpful, I'd be grateful for a positive review on Amazon.

8

Resources

leep. (2023, June 19). Cleveland Clinic. https://my.clevelandcl inic.org/health/body/12148-sleep-basics

Breus, M. (2023, July 19). *What happens during sleep.* Sleep Doctor. https://sleepdoctor.com/sleep-faqs/what-happens-when-you-sleep/

Sleep tips: 6 steps to better sleep. (2022, May 7). Mayo Clinic. https://www .mayoclinic.org/healthy-lifestyle/adult-health/in-depth/sleep/art-200 48379

Centers for Disease Control and Prevention. (2022, September 14). *CDC - How Much Sleep Do I Need? - Sleep and Sleep Disorders.* CDC; CDC. https://w ww.cdc.gov/sleep/about_sleep/how_much_sleep.html

CDC. (2023, August 1). *Benefits of Physical Activity.* Centers for Disease Control and Prevention. https://cdc.gov/physicalactivity/basics/pa-health/index.htm

British Heart Foundation. (2017, April 3). *What happens inside your body*

when you exercise? [Video]. YouTube.
https://www.youtube.com/watch?v=wWGulLAa0O0

Harvard Health. (2020, July 7). *Exercising to relax.* https://www.health.h
arvard.edu/staying-healthy/exercising-to-relax

Exercise: 7 benefits of regular physical activity. (2023, August 26). Mayo
Clinic. https://www.mayoclinic.org/healthy-lifestyle/fitness/in-depth/
exercise/art-20048389

Four Types of Exercise Can Improve Your Health and Physical Ability.
(n.d.). National Institute on Aging. Retrieved December 30, 2023, from
https://www.nia.nih.gov/health/exercise-and-physical-activity/four-t
ypes-exercise-can-improve-your-health-and-physical#balance

Harvard Health. (2017, February 6). *How it's made: Cholesterol production
in your body.* https://www.health.harvard.edu/heart-health/how-its-m
ade-cholesterol-production-in-your-body

Bergland, C. (2022, November 4). *What is ATP?* Verywell Health. https://w
ww.verywellhealth.com/atp-6374347

Eufic. (2019, December 16). *What are Proteins and What is Their Function
in the Body?* Eufic.org.
https://www.eufic.org/en/whats-in-food/article/what-are-proteins-a
nd-what-is-their-function-in-the-body

National Institutes of Health. (2022, July 18). *Office of Dietary Supplements
- Omega-3 Fatty Acids.* Nih.gov.
https://ods.od.nih.gov/factsheets/Omega3FattyAcids-Consumer/

Thorpe, M., MD PhD. (2023, July 3). *Healthy Fats vs. Unhealthy Fats: What You Need to Know.* Healthline. https://www.healthline.com/nutrition/healthy-vs-unhealthy-fats

Cronkleton, E. (2023, November 8). *Why is vitamin B complex important, and where do I get it?* Healthline. https://www.healthline.com/health/food-nutrition/vitamin-b-complex#foods-to-eat

CDC. (2022, August 23). *Potassium and Sodium.* Centers for Disease Control and Prevention. https://cdc.gov/salt/potassium.htm

Mind Tools . (2023). *SMART Goals.* Mind Tools. https://www.mindtools.com/a4wo118/smart-goals

Website, N. (2023, March 23). *8 tips for healthy eating.* nhs.uk. https://www.nhs.uk/live-well/eat-well/how-to-eat-a-balanced-diet/eight-tips-for-healthy-eating/

Rdn, A. B. M. (2023, February 6). *25 simple tips to make your diet healthier.* Healthline. https://www.healthline.com/nutrition/healthy-eating-tips
The Sunny Science of why we need sunlight – Morning sign out at UCI. (2021, August 4). https://sites.uci.edu/morningsignout/2021/08/04/the-sunny-science-of-why-we-need-sunlight/
Modern life may cause sun exposure, skin pigmentation mismatch. (2013, February 13). ScienceDaily. https://www.sciencedaily.com/releases/2013/02/130217084323.htm

Dresden, D. (2020, November 4). *What to know about the health benefits of sunlight.* https://www.medicalnewstoday.com/articles/benefits-of-s

unlight#health-benefits

Scaccia, A. (2023, April 17). *Everything you need to know about Serotonin.* Healthline. https://www.healthline.com/health/mental-health/serotonin#functions

Sunlight and your health. (n.d.). WebMD. https://www.webmd.com/a-to-z-guides/ss/slideshow-sunlight-health-effects

Crna, R. N. M. (2019, April 1). *What are the benefits of sunlight?* Healthline. https://www.healthline.com/health/depression/benefits-sunlight#benefits

Byzak, A. (2021, May 7). *5 Ways the sun Impacts your Mental and Physical Health – Tri-City Medical Center.* Tri-City Medical Center. https://www.tricitymed.org/2018/08/5-ways-the-sun-impacts-your-mental-and-physical-health/

Care, G. U. (2022, April 20). *The ideal amount of sunlight for a safe and healthy body – Getwell Urgent care.* Getwell Urgent Care. https://urgentcaresouthaven.com/the-ideal-amount-of-sunlight-for-a-safe-and-healthy-body

Rivers, A. (2023, August 18). *The importance of social connection.* Mind-Wise. https://www.mindwise.org/blog/uncategorized/the-importance-of-social-connection/

CDC. (2023a, May 8). *How Does Social Connectedness Affect Health?* Centers for Disease Control and Prevention. https://cdc.gov/emotional-wellbeing/social-connectedness/affect-health.htm

Services, D. of H. & H. (n.d.). *Strong relationships, strong health.* Www.betterhealth.vic.gov.au. Retrieved December 30, 2023, from https://betterh ealth.vic.gov.au/health/healthyliving/Strong-relationships-strong-he alth#health-benefits-of-strong-relationships

Improving social connection is a public health priority. (2023, May 2). *https://www.apa.org.* https://www.apa.org/news/press/releases/2023/0 5/improving-social-connection

Seppala, E. (2023, March 23). *Connectedness & Health: The Science of Social Connection - The Center for Compassion and Altruism Research and Education.* The Center for Compassion and Altruism Research and Education. https://ccare.stanford.edu/uncategorized/connectedness-h ealth-the-science-of-social-connection-infographic/

Hawkley, L. C., & Cacioppo, J. T. (2010). Loneliness Matters: A Theoretical and Empirical Review of Consequences and Mechanisms. *Annals of Behavioral Medicine*, 40(2), 218–227. https://www.ncbi.nlm.nih.gov /pmc/articles/PMC3874845/

Olff, M., Frijling, J. L., Kubzansky, L. D., Bradley, B., Ellenbogen, M. A., Cardoso, C., Bartz, J. A., Yee, J. R., & Van Zuiden, M. (2013). The role of oxytocin in social bonding, stress regulation and mental health: An update on the moderating effects of context and interindividual differences. *Psychoneuroendocrinology*, 38(9), 1883–1894. https://d oi.org/10.1016/j.psyneuen.2013.06.019

Clear, J. (2018). Atomic Habits. Penguin Random House

Huberman, A. [ahuberman]. (2023, Aug 30). *The most important step toward robust mental & physical health is when we realize that no single protocol, program supplement.* X. https://twitter.com/hubermanlab/statu s/1696831015229051282

Eisenberger, N. I. (2012). The pain of social disconnection: examining the shared neural underpinnings of physical and social pain. *Nature Reviews Neuroscience*, 13(6), 421–434. https://doi.org/10.1038/nrn3231

Lieberman M. (2013). Social: Why Our Brains Are Wired to Connect. Crown Publishers/Random House.